The
New Mediterranean
Diet Collection

Healthy and Easy Recipes to Boost your Metabolism

Jude Barnes

Table of Contents

Wild Rice Soup and Creamy Chicken

Preparation Time:

5 minutes

Cooking Time:

18 minutes

Servings: 8

Ingredients:

- 4 cups chicken broth
- 2 cups water
- 2 half-cooked and boneless chicken breast, grated
- 1 pack long-grain fast-cooking rice with a spice pack
- 1/2 teaspoon salt
- 1/2 teaspoon ground black pepper
- 3/4 cup flour
- 1/2 cup butter
- 2 cups thick cream

Directions:

1. Combine broth, water, and chicken in a large saucepan over medium heat.
2. Bring to a boil; stir in the rice, and save the seasoning package.
3. Cover and remove from heat.

4. Merge the flour with salt and pepper. Using a medium-sized pan, melt some butter over medium heat.

5. Stir the contents of the herb bag until the mixture bubbles.

6. Reduce the heat and add the flour mixture to the tablespoon to form a roux.

7. Stir the cream little by little until it is completely absorbed and smooth.

8. Bake until thick for 5 minutes.

9. Add the cream mixture to the stock and rice—cook over medium heat for 10 to 15 minutes.

Nutrition: Calories: 462 Fat: 36.5 g Carbohydrates: 22.6 g Protein: 12 g

Best Spanish rice

Preparation Time:

10 minutes

Cooking Time:

20 minutes

Servings: 5

Ingredients:

- 2 tablespoons oil
- 2 tablespoons chopped onion
- 1 1/2 cups uncooked white rice
- 2 cups chicken broth
- 1 cup chunky salsa

Directions:

1. Heat the oil and stir the onion and cook until tender, about 5 minutes.
2. Mix the rice in a pan, stirring often. When the rice starts to brown, stir in the chicken stock and salsa.
3. Lower the heat, cover, and simmer for 20 minutes until the liquid is absorbed.

Nutrition: Calories: 286 Fat: 6.2 g Carbohydrates: 50.9 g Protein: 5.7 g

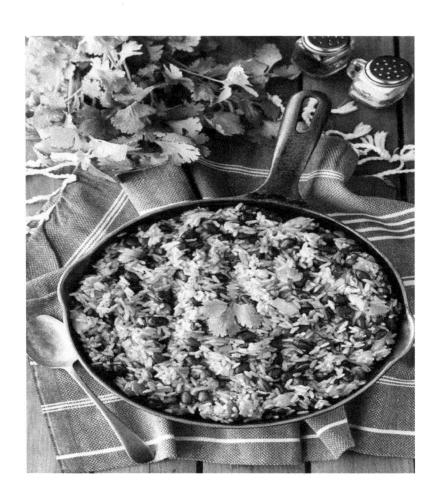

Classic Rice Pilaf

Preparation Time:

10 minutes

Cooking Time:

20 minutes

Servings: 6

Ingredients:

- 2 tablespoons butter
- 2 tablespoons olive oil
- 1/2 onion, minced
- 2 cups long-grain white rice
- 3 cups chicken broth
- 1 1/2 teaspoons of salt
- 1 pinch of saffron (optional)
- 1/4 teaspoon of cayenne pepper

Directions:

1. Preheat the oven.
2. Heat the butter until it reaches a liquid form.
3. Attach the melted butter and olive oil to a large saucepan over medium heat.
4. Add and cook the minced onion, continuously stirring until the onion is

light brown in color, 7 to 8 minutes. Remove from the heat.

5. Combine rice and onion in a 9x13-inch baking dish on a baking sheet. Mix well to cover the rice.

6. Mix chicken broth, salt, saffron, and cayenne pepper in a pan.

7. Pour the chicken stock mixture over the rice in the casserole and mix. Pour the mixture evenly over the bottom of the pan. Cover firmly with sturdy aluminum foil.

8. Bake and remove from the oven and leave under cover for 10 minutes.

9. Remove the aluminum foil and stir with a fork to separate the rice grains.

Nutrition: Calories: 312 Fat: 9.1 g Carbohydrates: 51.7 g Protein: 5 g

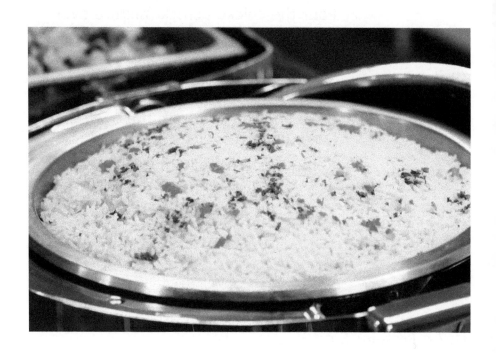

Sarah's Rice Pilaf

Preparation Time:

10 minutes

Cooking Time:

20 minutes

Servings: 4

Ingredients:

- 2 tablespoons butter
- 1/2 cup orzo
- 1/2 cup diced onion
- 2 cloves finely chopped garlic
- 1/2 cup uncooked white rice
- 2 cups chicken broth

Directions:

1. Dissolve the butter in a frying pan. Boil and mix the orzo pasta golden brown.
2. Stir in the onion and cook until it is transparent, then add the garlic and cook for 1 minute.
3. Stir in the rice and chicken broth. Lower the heat until the rice is soft and the liquid is absorbed for 20 to 25 minutes.
4. Detach from heat and let stand for 5 minutes, and then stir with a fork.

Nutrition: Calories: 244 Carbohydrates: 40 g Protein: 5.9 g

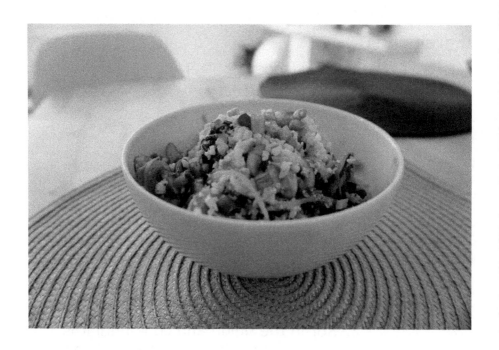

Homemade Fried Rice

Preparation Time:

10 minutes

Cooking Time:

23 minutes

Servings: 8

Ingredients:

- 1 1/2 cup uncooked white rice
- 3 tablespoons sesame oil
- 1 small onion, minced
- 1 clove garlic, minced
- 1 cup peeled shrimp
- 1/2 cup diced ham
- 1 cup chopped cooked chicken fillet
- 2 celery stalks, minced
- 2 carrots, peeled and diced
- 1 green pepper, minced
- 1/2 cup of green peas
- 1 beaten egg
- 1/4 cup soy sauce

Directions:

1. Cook the rice.
2. While cooking the rice, heat a wok or large frying pan over medium heat.
3. Pour in the sesame oil and sauté in the onion until golden brown.
4. Add the garlic, shrimp, ham, and chicken.
5. Cook until the shrimp are pink.
6. Reduce the heat and stir in celery, carrot, green pepper, and peas.
7. Bake until the vegetables are soft.
8. Whip in the beaten egg and cook.
9. When the rice is cooked, merge it with the vegetables and soy sauce.

Nutrition: Calories: 236 Fat: 8.4 g Carbohydrates: 26.4 g; Protein: 13 g

Cranberry Rice

Preparation Time:

5 minutes

Cooking Time:

23 minutes

Servings: 6

Ingredients:

- 2/3 cup uncooked brown rice
- 1 1/2 cups water
- 2 tablespoons canned cranberry sauce
- 1/2 cup of dried cranberries
- Salt and black pepper to taste
- 1/4 cup chopped pecans

Directions:

1. Cook the rice.
2. Squash the cranberry sauce in a small bowl with a fork and mix with the brown rice.
3. Put the dried cranberries in a bowl microwave and cook them on high heat in the microwave for about 30 seconds.
4. Stir the cranberries into the rice.
5. Season it with salt and black pepper; sprinkle with pecans.

Nutrition: Calories: 129 Fat: 3.7 g Carbohydrates: 23.4 g Protein: 1.6 g

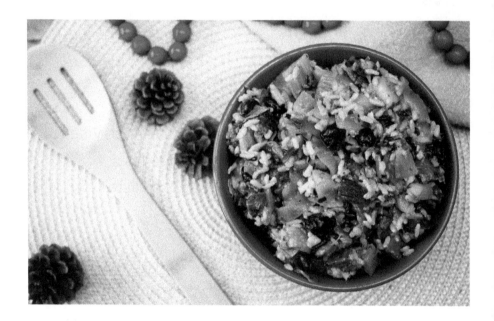

Kickin' Rice

Preparation Time:

10 minutes

Cooking Time:

23 minutes

Servings: 6

Ingredients:

- 1 tablespoon vegetable oil
- 1 cup long-grain white rice
- 1 can chopped green peppers
- 1 teaspoon ground black pepper
- 2 cups chicken broth

Directions:

1. Heat the vegetable oil. Stir the rice in hot oil.
2. Add the green peppers and keep cooking until the rice starts to turn a little brown, 2 to 3 minutes.
3. Season the rice with pepper.
4. Whisk the stock into the pan; bring to a boil.
5. Reduce the heat to low, cover the pan and cook until the broth has been absorbed.

Nutrition: Calories: 83 Fat: 2.6 g Carbohydrates: 13 g
Protein: 1.9 g

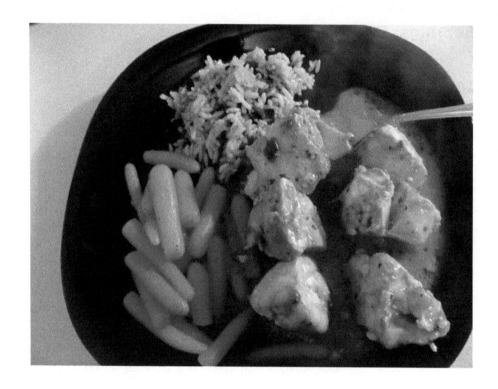

Garlic Rice

Preparation Time:

5 minutes

Cooking Time:

15 minutes

Servings: 6

Ingredients:

- 2 tablespoons vegetable oil
- 1 1/2 tablespoons chopped garlic
- 2 tablespoons ground pork
- 4 cups cooked white rice
- 1 1/2 teaspoons of garlic salt
- Ground black pepper to taste

Directions:

1. Heat the oil.
2. Attach the garlic and ground pork.
3. Boil and stir until garlic is golden brown.
4. Stir in cooked white rice and season with garlic, salt, and pepper.
5. Bake and stir until the mixture is hot and well mixed for about 3 minutes.

Nutrition: Calories: 83 Fat: 2.6 g Carbohydrates: 13 g Protein: 1.9 g

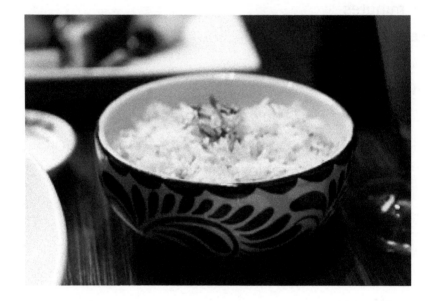

Sweet Rice

Preparation Time:

10 minutes

Cooking Time:

15 minutes

Servings: 6

Ingredients:

- 1 cup uncooked long-grain white rice
- 2 tablespoons unsalted butter
- 2 cups water
- 2 cups whole milk
- 1 tablespoon all-purpose flour
- 1/3 cup white sugar
- 1 egg
- 1 1/2 teaspoon vanilla extract
- 1 cup whole milk
- 2/3 cup thick cream
- 1/2 cup raisins (optional)
- 1/2 teaspoon ground cinnamon

Directions:

1. Add rice and butter to water in a large saucepan and bring to boil over high heat.

2. Mix 2 cups of milk, flour, sugar, egg, and vanilla extract in a bowl and pour the milk mixture over the cooked rice.

3. Mix and simmer for 15 minutes over low heat.

4. Stir in 1 cup of whole milk, cream, raisins, and cinnamon until it is well mixed.

Nutrition: Calories: 418 Fat: 18.6 g Carbohydrates: 55 g Protein: 8.6 g

Gourmet Mushroom Risotto

Preparation Time:

20 minutes

Cooking Time:

15 minutes

Servings: 6

Ingredients:

- 1 kg Portobello mushrooms, minced
- 1 pound of white mushrooms, minced
- 2 shallots, diced
- 3 tablespoons olive oil, divided
- 1 1/2 cup Arborio rice
- Salt and black pepper to taste
- 1/2 cup dry white wine
- 4 tablespoons butter
- 3 tablespoons finely chopped chives
- 6 cups chicken broth, divided
- 1/3 cup Parmesan cheese

Directions:

1. Heat the broth over low heat.
2. Attach 2 tablespoons of olive oil in a huge saucepan over medium heat. Whip in the mushrooms and cook until

soft. Now remove the mushrooms and their liquid and set them aside.

3. Attach 1 tablespoon of olive oil in the pan and stir in the shallots.

4. Cook for 1 minute and add the rice, stirring, to cover with foil for about 2 minutes.

5. When the rice has turned a pale golden color, pour the wine constantly, stirring until the wine is completely absorbed.

6. Add 1/2 cup of rice broth and mix until the broth has been absorbed.

7. Continue to add 1/2 cup of broth at a time, constantly stirring.

8. Then detach from the heat and stir in the mushrooms with their liquid, butter, chives, and Parmesan cheese.

9. Season with salt and pepper.

Nutrition: Calories: 418 Fat: 18.6 g Carbohydrates: 55 g Protein: 8.6 g

John's Beans and Rice

Preparation Time:

20 minutes

Cooking Time:

15 minutes

Servings: 6

Ingredients:

- 1 pound dry red beans
- 1 tablespoon of vegetable oil
- 12 grams of Andouille sausage, diced
- 1 cup finely chopped onion
- 3/4 cup chopped celery
- 3/4 cup poblano peppers
- 4 cloves of garlic, minced
- 2 pints of chicken broth or more if necessary
- 1 smoked ham shank
- 2 bay leaves
- 1 teaspoon dried thyme
- 1/2 teaspoon cayenne pepper
- 1 teaspoon freshly ground black pepper
- 2 tablespoons chopped green onion,
- 4 cups cooked white rice

Directions:

1. Bring the beans in a large container and cover them with a few centimeters of cold water; soak overnight.

2. Drain and rinse.

3. Heat the oil and cook and stir sausage in hot oil for 5 to 7 minutes.

4. Stir in onion, celery, and poblano peppers in sausage; cook and stir until the vegetables soften and start to become transparent, 5 to 10 minutes.

5. Add the garlic to the sausage mixture; cook and stir until fragrant, about 1 minute.

6. Stir in brown beans, chicken broth, ham shank, bay leaf, black pepper, thyme, cayenne pepper, and the sausage mixture; bring to a boil, reduce the heat, and stir occasionally, for an hour and a half.

7. Season with salt and simmer until the beans are soft, the meat is soft, and the desired consistency is achieved, 1 1/2 to 2 hours more.

8. Season with salt.

9. Put the rice in bowls, place the red bean mixture on the rice, and garnish with green onions.

Nutrition: Calories: 542 Fat: 25 g Carbohydrates: 36 g
Protein: 8.6 g

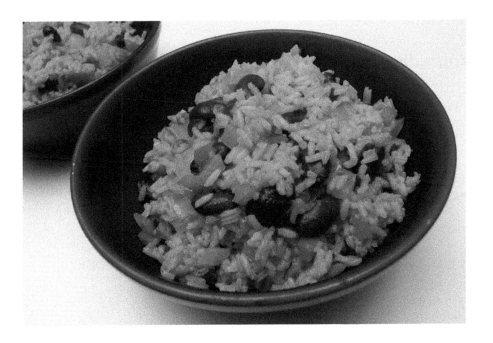

Creamy Chicken and Wild Rice Soup

Preparation Time:

10 minutes

Cooking Time:

15 minutes

Servings: 8

Ingredients:

- 2 cups water
- 4 cups chicken broth
- 2 boneless chicken fillet and cooked, grated
- 1 pack long-grain fast-cooking rice with a spice pack
- 1/2 teaspoon salt
- 1/2 teaspoon ground black pepper
- 3/4 cup all-purpose flour
- 1/2 cup butter
- 2 cups thick cream

Directions:

1. Combine broth, water, and chicken in a large saucepan over medium heat.
2. Bring to a boil; stir in the rice, and save the seasoning package.
3. Cover and remove from heat.

4. Merge salt, pepper, and flour. Dissolve the butter.

5. Stir the contents of the herb bag until the mixture bubbles.

6. Reduce the heat and add the flour mixture to a tablespoon to form a roux.

7. Stir the cream little by little until it is completely absorbed and smooth. Bake until thick, 5 minutes.

8. Add the cream mixture to the stock and rice.

9. Cook over medium heat for 10 to 15 minutes.

Nutrition: Calories: 426 Fat: 35 g Carbohydrates: 41 g Protein: 8.6 g

Carrot Rice

Preparation Time:

5 minutes

Cooking Time:

15 minutes

Servings: 6

Ingredients:

- 2 cups water
- 1 cube chicken broth
- 1 grated carrot
- 1 cup uncooked long-grain rice

Directions:

1. Boil the water and lace in the bouillon cube and let it dissolve.
2. Stir in the carrots and rice and bring to a boil again.
3. Lower the heats, cover, and simmer for 20 minutes.
4. Remove from heat and leave under cover for 5 minutes.

Nutrition: Calories: 125 Fat: 41 g Carbohydrates: 32 g Protein: 16 g

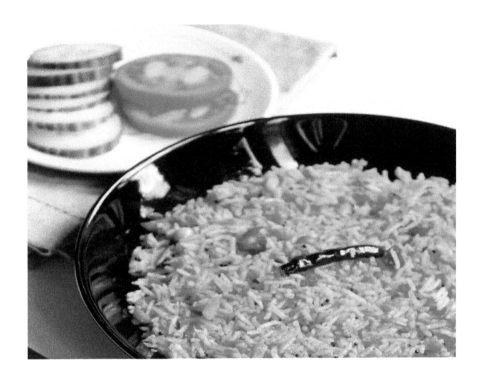

Rice Sauce

Preparation Time:

5 minutes

Cooking Time:

15 minutes

Servings: 6

Ingredients:

- 3 cups cooked rice
- 1 1/4 cup grated Monterey Jack cheese, divided
- 1 cup canned or frozen corn
- 1/2 cup of milk
- 1/3 cup of sour cream
- 1/2 cup chopped green onions

Directions:

1. Preheat the oven.
2. Combine rice, a cup of cheese, corn, milk, sour cream, and green onions in a medium-sized bowl.
3. Put in a 1-liter baking dish and sprinkle the rest of the cheese over it.
4. Bake until the cheese is dissolved and the dish is hot.

Nutrition: Calories: 110 Fat: 32 g Carbohydrates: 54 g
Protein: 12 g

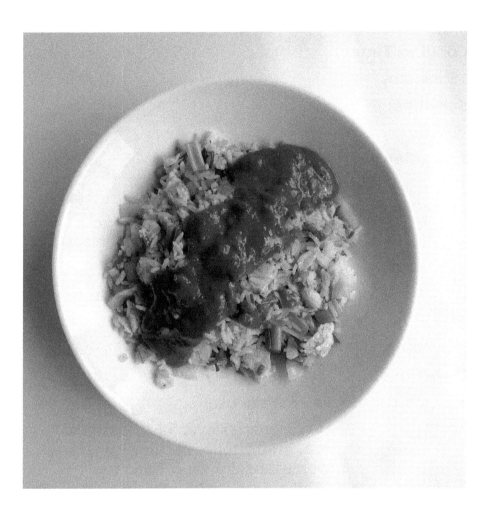

Brown Rice

Preparation Time:

5 minutes

Cooking Time:

15 minutes

Servings: 4

Ingredients:

- 1 1/2 cup white rice
- 1 beef broth
- 1 condensed soup of French onions
- 1/4 cup melted butter
- 1 tablespoon Worcestershire sauce
- 1 tablespoon dried basil leaves

Directions:

1. Preheat the oven.
2. In a 2-quarter oven dish, combine rice, broth, soup, butter, Worcestershire sauce, and basil.
3. Prepare for 1 hour, stirring after 30 minutes.

Nutrition: Calories: 425 Fat: 33 g Carbohydrates: 21 g Protein: 12 g

Rice Lasagna

Preparation Time:

20 minutes

Cooking Time:

15 minutes

Servings: 8

Ingredients:

- 1 pound ground beef
- Spaghetti sauce
- 3 cups cooked rice, cooled
- 1/2 teaspoon garlic powder
- 2 eggs
- 3/4 cup grated Parmesan cheese
- 2 1/4 cup grated mozzarella cheese
- 2 cups of cottage cheese

Directions:

1. Preheat the oven to 190°C.
2. Fry and stir the meat in a hot pan until golden brown and crumbly, 5 to 7 minutes; drain the Fat: and discard it.
3. Add the spaghetti sauce and garlic powder.
4. Mix the rice, eggs, and 1/4 cup Parmesan cheese in a bowl.

5. Mix 2 cups mozzarella, cottage cheese, and 1/4 cup Parmesan cheese in another bowl.

6. Set half of the rice mixture in a 3-liter baking dish, followed by the cheese mixture and half of the meat sauce. Repeat the layers.

7. Sprinkle 1/4 cup Parmesan cheese and 1/4 cup mozzarella on the last layer of meat sauce.

8. Until the cheese is dissolved and the sauce is bubbling 20 to 25 minutes.

Nutrition: Calories: 461 Fat: 31 g Carbohydrates: 11 g Protein: 13 g

Rice Milk

Preparation Time:

5 minutes

Cooking Time:

15 minutes

Servings: 4

Ingredients:

- 4 cups cold water
- 1 cup cooked rice
- 1 teaspoon vanilla extract (optional)

Directions:

1. Combine water, cooked rice, and vanilla extract in a blender; blend until smooth, about 3 minutes.
2. Chill before serving.

Nutrition: Calories: 54 Fat: 32 g Carbohydrates: 21 g Protein: 26 g

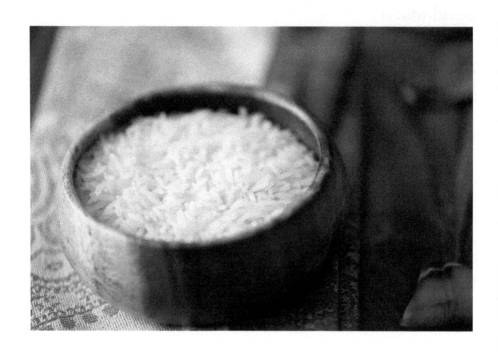

Breakfast Salad from Grains and Fruits

Preparation Time:

5 minutes

Cooking Time:

20 minutes

Servings: 6

Ingredients:

- 1/4 teaspoon salt
- 3/4 cup bulgur
- 3/4 cup quick-cooking brown rice
- 1 8-oz low-fat vanilla yogurt
- 1 cup raisins
- 1 Granny Smith apple
- 1 orange
- 1 red delicious apple
- 3 cups water

Directions:

1. On high fire, place a large pot and bring water to a boil.
2. Add bulgur and rice. Slow down the fire to a simmer and cook for ten minutes while covered.
3. Turn off fire, set aside for 2 minutes while covered.

4. On a baking sheet, transfer and evenly spread grains to cool.

5. Meanwhile, peel oranges and cut them into sections. Chop and core apples.

6. Once the grains are cool, transfer to a large serving bowl along with fruits.

7. Add yogurt and mix well to coat.

8. Serve and enjoy.

Nutrition: Calories: 48.6 Carbs: 23.9 g Protein: 3.7 g Fat: 1.1 g

Puttanesca Style Bucatini

Preparation Time:

5 minutes

Cooking Time:

40 minutes

Servings: 4

Ingredients:

- 1 tablespoon capers, rinsed
- 1 teaspoon coarsely chopped fresh oregano
- 1 teaspoon finely chopped garlic
- 1/8 teaspoon salt
- 12-oz bucatini pasta
- 2 cups coarsely chopped canned no-salt-added whole peeled tomatoes with their juice
- 3 tablespoons extra virgin olive oil, divided
- 4 anchovy fillets, chopped
- 8 black Kalamata olives, pitted and sliced into slivers

Directions:

1. Cook bucatini pasta according to package directions.
2. Drain, keep warm and set aside.

45

3. On medium fire, place a large nonstick saucepan and heat 2 tablespoons of oil.

4. Sauté the anchovy until it starts to disintegrate.

5. Add garlic and sauté for 15 seconds.

6. Add tomatoes, sauté for 15 to 20 minutes, or until no longer watery. Season with 1/8 teaspoon salt.

7. Add oregano, capers, and olives.

8. Add pasta, sautéing until heated through.

9. To serve, drizzle pasta with remaining olive oil and enjoy.

Nutrition: Calories: 207.4 Carbs: 31 g Protein: 5.1 g Fat: 7 g

Sausage and Bean Casserole

Preparation Time:

15 minutes

Cooking Time:

45 minutes

Servings: 4

Ingredients:

- 1 pound Italian sausages
- 1 can cannellini beans, drained
- 1 carrot, chopped
- 2 tablespoons olive oil
- 1 onion, chopped
- 2 garlic cloves, minced
- 1 teaspoon paprika
- 1 can tomatoes in juice, chopped
- 1/4 cup chopped fresh parsley
- 1 celery stalk, chopped
- Salt and black pepper to taste

Directions:

1. Preheat oven to 350°F.
2. Heat the olive oil and sauté onion, garlic, celery, and carrot for 3-4 minutes, stirring often until softened.

3. Add in sausages and cook for another 3 minutes, turning occasionally.

4. Stir in paprika for 30 seconds. Turn the heat off and mix in tomatoes, beans, salt, and pepper.

5. Pour into a baking dish and bake for 30 minutes.

6. Serve topped with parsley.

Nutrition: Calories: 862 Fat: 43.6 g Carbs: 76.2 g Protein: 43.4 g

Hot Vegetarian Two-Bean Cassoulet

Preparation Time:

15 minutes

Cooking Time:

40 minutes

Servings: 4

Ingredients:

- 1 cup canned pinto beans, drained
- 1 cup canned can kidney beans, drained
- 2 red bell peppers, seeded and chopped
- 1 onion, chopped
- 1 celery stalk, chopped
- 2 garlic cloves, minced
- 1 can crushed tomatoes
- 2 tablespoons olive oil
- 1 tablespoon red pepper flakes
- 1 teaspoon ground cumin
- Salt and black pepper to taste
- 1/4 teaspoon ground coriander

Directions:

1. Heat the olive oil and sauté bell peppers, celery, garlic, and onion for 5 minutes until tender.

2. Stir in ground cumin, ground coriander, salt, and pepper for 1 minute. Pour in beans, tomatoes, and red pepper flakes.

3. Bring to a boil, then decrease the heat and simmer for another 20 minutes.

4. Serve immediately.

Nutrition: Calories: 361 Fat: 8.4 g Carbs: 55.7 g Protein: 17.1 g

Moroccan Spiced Couscous

Preparation Time:

15 minutes

Cooking Time:

25 minutes

Servings: 4

Ingredients:

- 1 cup instant couscous
- 2 tablespoons dried apricots, chopped
- 2 tablespoons dried sultanas
- 2 tablespoons olive oil
- 1/2 onion, minced
- 1 orange, juiced, and zested
- 1/4 teaspoon paprika
- 1/4 teaspoon turmeric
- 1/2 teaspoon garlic powder
- 1/2 teaspoon ground cumin
- 1/4 teaspoon ground cinnamon
- Salt and black pepper to taste

Directions:

1. Heat the oil and sauté onion for 3 minutes.
2. Add in orange juice, orange zest, garlic powder, cumin, salt, paprika, turmeric,

cinnamon, black pepper, and 2 cups of
water.

3. Stir in apricots, couscous, and
sultanas.

4. Detach from the heat and let it sit for
5 minutes.

5. Fluff the couscous using a fork.

6. Serve.

Nutrition: Calories: 246 Fat: 7.4 g Carbs: 41.8 g
Protein: 5.2 g

Bulgur Tabbouleh

Preparation Time:

15 minutes

Cooking Time:

30 minutes

Servings: 4

Ingredients:

- 8 cherry tomatoes, quartered
- 1 cucumber, peeled and chopped
- 1 cup bulgur, rinsed
- 4 scallions, chopped
- 1/2 cup fresh parsley, chopped
- 1 lemon, juiced
- 1/4 cup extra-virgin olive oil
- Salt and black pepper to taste

Directions:

1. Set the bulgur in a large pot with plenty of salted water, cover, and boil for 13-15 minutes.
2. Drain and let it cool completely.
3. Add scallions, tomatoes, cucumber, and parsley to the cooled bulgur and mix to combine.

4. Merge the lemon juice, olive oil, salt, and pepper.

5. Pour the dressing over the bulgur mixture and toss to combine.

6. Serve chilled.

Nutrition: Calories: 291 Fat: 13.7 g Carbs: 40.4 g Protein: 7.4 g

Parmesan and Collard Green Oats

Preparation Time:

15 minutes

Cooking Time:

15 minutes

Servings: 4

Ingredients:

- 2 cups collard greens, torn into pieces
- 1/2 cup black olives
- 1 cup rolled oats
- 2 tomatoes, diced
- 2 spring onions, chopped
- 1 teaspoon garlic powder
- 1/2 teaspoon hot paprika
- A pinch of salt
- 2 tablespoons fresh parsley, chopped
- 1 tablespoon lemon juice
- 2 tablespoons olive oil
- 1/2 cup Parmesan cheese, grated

Directions:

1. Attach 2 cups of water in a pot over medium heat.
2. Bring to a boil, then lower the heat, and add the rolled oats.

3. Cook for 4-5 minutes.

4. Mix in tomatoes, spring onions, hot paprika, garlic powder, salt, collard greens, black olives, parsley, lemon juice, and olive oil.

5. Cook for another 5 minutes.

6. Spread into bowls and top with Parmesan cheese.

7. Serve warm.

Nutrition: Calories: 192 Fat: 11.2 g Carbs: 19.8 g Protein: 5.3 g

Italian Barley with Artichoke Hearts

Preparation Time:

15 minutes

Cooking Time:

50 minutes

Servings: 4

Ingredients:

- 1 cup pearl barley
- 1/2 cup artichoke hearts, chopped
- 2 tablespoons grated Parmesan cheese
- 1 bay leaf
- 1 fresh cilantro sprig
- 1 fresh thyme sprig
- 2 tablespoons olive oil
- 1 onion, chopped
- 1 tablespoon Italian seasoning
- 3 garlic cloves, minced
- 1 cup chicken broth
- 1 lemon, zested
- Salt and black pepper to taste

Directions:

1. Place barley, cilantro, bay leaf, and thyme in a pot over medium heat and cover with water.

2. Parboil, then lower the heat and simmer for 25 minutes. Drain; discard the bay leaf, rosemary, and thyme and reserve.

3. Heat the olive oil and sauté onion, artichoke, and Italian seasoning for 5 minutes.

4. Add garlic and stir-fry for 40 seconds. Whisk in some broth and cook until the liquid is absorbed, then add more, and keep stirring until it is absorbed again.

5. Mix in lemon zest, salt, pepper, and cheese and stir for 2 minutes until the cheese has melted.

6. Pour over the barley and serve.

Nutrition: Calories: 325 Fat: 12 g Carbs: 45.4 g Protein: 11.8 g

Cole Slaw

Preparation Time:

10 minutes

Cooking Time:

0 minutes

Servings: 1

Ingredients:

- Coleslaw mix, tri-color,
- 1 1/2 cups - carrots should be taken out, (3 Greens)
- Apple cider vinegar,
- 2 tsp., (1/6 Condiment)
- Olive oil, 1 tsp., (1 Healthy Fat)
- Stevia, 1/2 packet (1/2 Condiment)

Directions:

In a medium bowl, mix all the ingredients and enjoy.

Nutrition: Energy (calories): 32 kcal--Protein: 0.61 g--Fat: 0.66 g --Carbohydrates: 6.44 g

Quick and Easy Egg Salad

Preparation Time:

10 minutes

Cooking Time:

0 minutes

Servings: 2

Ingredients:

- Hard-boiled Eggs, 6 (2 Leans)
- Dijon mustard,
- 2 tsp. (2 Condiments)
- Greek yogurt, plain, low fat, (2 Condiments)
- Finely chopped fresh chives,
- 2 tbsp. (1/2 Condiment)
- Salt, 1/4 tsp., (1 Condiment)
- Paprika, 1/4 tsp., (1/2 Condiment)
- Finely chopped, dill pickle spear, 2, (1 Optional Snack)

Directions:

1. In a medium-sized bowl, put peeled and chopped eggs.
2. Add Greek yogurt, Dijon mustard, salt, chives, pickles, and paprika.
3. Mix with care until it is fully combined.

4. The leftovers can be refrigerated for up to 3 days.

Nutrition: Energy (calories): 43 kcal Protein: 2.89 g Fat: 3.02 g Carbohydrates: 1.19 g

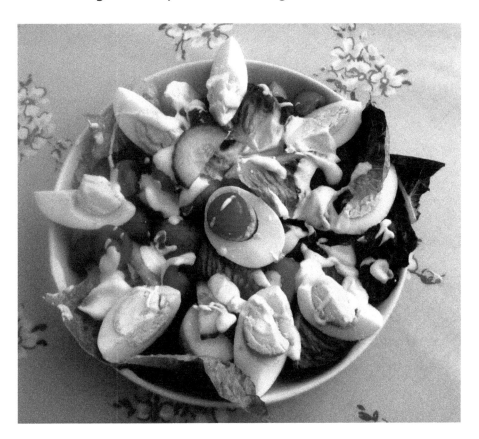

High-Protein Salad

Preparation Time:

15 minutes

Cooking Time:

16 minutes

Servings: 4

Ingredients:

- 4 (6-oz.) boneless, skinless chicken breast halves
- Salt and freshly ground black pepper, to taste
- 2 tbsp. olive oil
- 1/2 C. cherry tomatoes, halved
- 3 C. fresh baby greens
- 3 C. lettuce, torn

Directions:

1. Season each chicken breast half with salt and black pepper evenly.
2. Place chicken over a rack set in a rimmed baking sheet. Refrigerate for at least 30 minutes.
3. Remove from refrigerator and with paper towels, pat dry the chicken breasts.
4. In a 12-inch skillet, heat the oil over medium-low heat.

5. Place the chicken breast halves, smooth-side down, and cook for about 9-10 minutes, without moving.

6. Flip the chicken breasts and cook for about 6 minutes or until cooked through.

7. Remove the skillet from heat and let the chicken stand in the pan for about 3 minutes.

8. Divide greens, lettuce, and tomatoes onto serving plates.

9. Top each plate with 1 breasts half and serves.

Nutrition: Calories per serving: 276; Carbohydrates: 2.6g; Protein: 38.7g; Fat: 10g; Sugar: 1.3g; Sodium: 146mg; Fiber: 0.8g

Refreshing Dinner Salad

Preparation Time:

15 minutes

Cooking Time:

0 minutes

Servings: 4

Ingredients:

- For Vinaigrette:
- 2 tbsp. apple cider vinegar
- 2 tbsp. extra-virgin olive oil
- Salt and freshly ground black pepper, to taste
- For Salad:
- 2 C. cooked chicken, cubed
- 4 C. lettuce, torn
- 1 large apple, peeled, cored and chopped
- 1 C. fresh strawberries, hulled and sliced

Directions:

1. For vinaigrette: in a small bowl, add all ingredients and beat well.
2. For salad: in a large salad bowl, mix all ingredients.

3. Place vinaigrette over chicken mixture and toss to coat well.

4. Serve immediately.

Nutrition: Calories per serving: 215; Carbohydrates: 12g; Protein: 20.9g; Fat: 9.4g; Sugar: 8g; Sodium: 87mg; Fiber: 2.4g

Real Food Salad

Preparation Time:

15 minutes

Cooking Time:

0 minutes

Servings: 2

Ingredients:

- 6 oz. cooked wild salmon, chopped
- 1 C. cucumber, sliced
- 1 C. red bell pepper, seeded and sliced
- 1/2 C. grape tomatoes, quartered
- 1 tbsp. scallion green, chopped
- 1 C. lettuce, torn
- 1 C. fresh spinach, torn
- 2 tbsp. olive oil
- 2 tbsp. fresh lemon juice

Directions:

1. In a salad bowl, place all ingredients and gently toss to coat well.
2. Serve immediately.

Nutrition: Calories per serving: 279; Carbohydrates: 10g; Protein: 18.6g; Fat: 19.8g; Sugar: 5g; Sodium: 59mg; Fiber: 2.2g

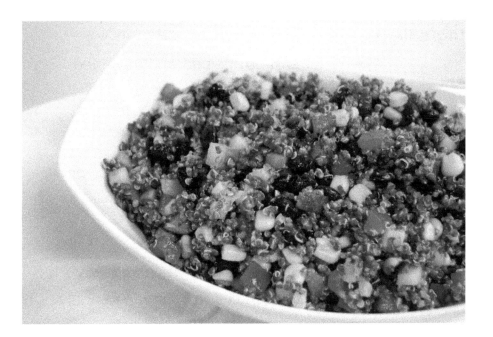

Light Entrée Salad

Preparation Time:

15 minutes

Cooking Time:

3 minutes

Servings: 4

Ingredients:

- 1 lb. shrimp, peeled and deveined
- 1 lemon, quartered
- 2 tbsp. olive oil
- 2 tsp. fresh lemon juice
- Salt and freshly ground black pepper, to taste
- 2 tomatoes, sliced
- 1/4 C. onion, sliced
- 1/4 C. green olives
- 1/4 C. fresh cilantro, chopped finely

Directions:

1. In a pan of lightly salted boiling water, add the quartered lemon.
2. Then, add the shrimp and cook for about 2-3 minutes or until pink and opaque.
3. With a slotted spoon, transfer the shrimp into a bowl of ice water to stop the cooking process.

4. Drain the shrimp completely and then pat dry with paper towels.

5. In a small bowl, add the oil, lemon juice, salt, and black pepper, and beat until well combined.

6. Divide the shrimp, tomato, onion, olives, and cilantro onto serving plates.

7. Drizzle with oil mixture and serve.

Nutrition: Calories per serving: 220; Carbohydrates: 5.8g; Protein: 26.2g; Fat: 4.5g; Sugar: 21g; Sodium: 393mg; Fiber: 1.3g

Marinated Tuna Steak

Preparation Time:

5 minutes

Cooking Time:

15-20 Minutes

Servings: 4

Ingredients:

- Olive oil (2 tbsp.)
- Orange juice (.25 cup)
- Soy sauce (.25 cup)
- Lemon juice (1 tbsp.)
- Fresh parsley (2 tbsp.)
- Garlic clove (1)
- Ground black pepper (.5 tsp.)
- Fresh oregano (.5 tsp.)
- Tuna steaks (4 - 4 oz. Steaks)

Directions:

1. Mince the garlic and chop the oregano and parsley.
2. In a glass container, mix the pepper, oregano, garlic, parsley, lemon juice, soy sauce, olive oil, and orange juice.
3. Warm the grill using the high heat setting. Grease the grate with oil.

4. Add to tuna steaks and cook for five to six minutes. Turn and baste with the marinated sauce.

5. Cook another five minutes or until it's the way you like it.

6. Discard the remaining marinade.

Nutrition: Calories: 200; Protein: 27.4 grams; Fat: 7.9 grams

Garlic And Shrimp Pasta

Preparation Time:

5 minutes

Cooking Time:

15 Minutes

Servings: 4

Ingredients:

- 6 ounces whole wheat spaghetti
- 12 ounces raw shrimp, peeled and deveined, cut into 1-inch pieces
- 1 bunch asparagus, trimmed
- 1 large bell pepper, thinly sliced
- 1 cup fresh peas
- 3 garlic cloves, chopped
- 1 and ¼ teaspoons kosher salt
- ½ and ½ cups non-fat plain yogurt
- 3 tablespoon lemon juice
- 1 tablespoon extra-virgin olive oil
- ½ teaspoon fresh ground black pepper
- ¼ cup pine nuts, toasted

Directions:

1. Take a large sized pot and bring water to a boil

2. Add your spaghetti and cook them for about minutes less than the directed package instruction

3. Add shrimp, bell pepper, asparagus and cook for about 2- 4 minutes until the shrimp are tender

4. Drain the pasta and the contents well

5. Take a large bowl and mash garlic until a paste form

6. Whisk in yogurt, parsley, oil, pepper and lemon juice into the garlic paste

7. Add pasta mix and toss well

8. Serve by sprinkling some pine nuts!

9. Enjoy!

Nutrition: Calories: 406; Fat: 22g; Carbohydrates: 28g; Protein: 26g

Paprika Butter Shrimps

Preparation Time:

5 minutes

Cooking Time:

30 Minutes

Servings: 2

Ingredients:

- ¼ tablespoon smoked paprika
- 1/8 cup sour cream
- ½ pound tiger shrimps
- 1/8 cup butter
- Salt and black pepper, to taste

Directions:

1. Preheat the oven to 390 degrees F and grease a baking dish.
2. Mix all the ingredients in a large bowl and transfer into the baking dish.
3. Place in the oven and bake for about 15 minutes.
4. Place paprika shrimp in a dish and set aside to cool for meal prepping.
5. Divide it in 2 containers and cover the lid.
6. Refrigerate for 1-2 days and reheat in microwave before serving.

Nutrition: Calories: 330; Carbohydrates: 1. Protein: 32.6g; Fat: 21.5g; Sugar: 0.2g; Sodium: 458mg

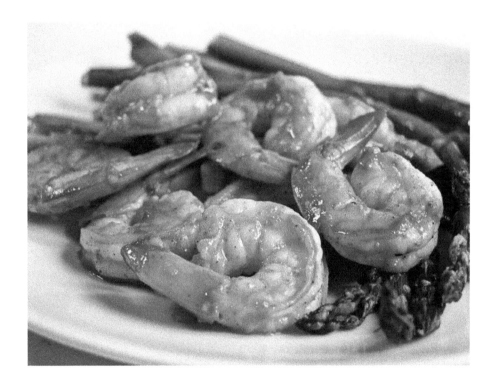

Mediterranean Avocado Salmon Salad

Preparation Time:

5 minutes

Cooking Time:

10 Minutes

Servings: 4

Ingredients:

- 1 lb skinless salmon fillets

Marinade/Dressing:

- 3 tbsp olive oil
- 2 tbsp lemon juice fresh, squeezed
- 1 tbsp red wine vinegar, optional
- 1 tbsp fresh chopped parsley
- 2 tsp garlic minced
- 1 tsp dried oregano
- 1 tsp salt
- Cracked pepper, to taste

Salad:

- 4 cups Romaine (or Cos) lettuce leaves, washed and dried
- 1 large cucumber, diced
- 2 Roma tomatoes, diced
- 1 red onion, sliced

- 1 avocado, sliced
- 1/2 cup feta cheese crumbled
- 1/3 cup pitted Kalamata olives or black olives, sliced
- Lemon wedges to serve

Directions:

1. In a jug, whisk together the olive oil, lemon juice, red wine vinegar, chopped parsley; garlic minced, oregano, salt and pepper
2. Pour out half of the marinade into a large, shallow dish; refrigerate the remaining marinade to use as the dressing
3. Coat the salmon in the rest of the marinade
4. Place a skillet pan or grill over medium-high, add 1 tbsp oil and sear salmon on both sides until crispy and cooked through
5. Allow the salmon to cool
6. Distribute the salmon among the containers, store in the fridge for 2-3 days
7. To Serve: Prepare the salad by placing the romaine lettuce, cucumber, roma tomatoes, red onion, avocado, feta cheese, and olives in a large salad bowl.

8. Reheat the salmon in the microwave for 30seconds to 1 minute or until heated through.

9. Slice the salmon and arrange over salad. Drizzle the salad with the remaining untouched dressing, serve with lemon wedges.

Nutrition: Calories: 411; Carbs: 12g; Total Fat: 27g; Protein: 28g

Beet Kale Salad

Preparation Time:

5 minutes

Cooking Time:

50 Minutes

Servings: 6

Ingredients:

- 1 bunch of kale, washed and dried, ribs removed, chopped
- 6 pieces washed beets, peeled and dried and cut into ½ inches
- ½ teaspoon dried rosemary
- ½ teaspoon garlic powder
- salt
- pepper
- olive oil
- ¼ medium red onion, thinly sliced
- 1-2 tablespoons slivered almonds, toasted
- ¼ cup olive oil
- Juice of 1½ lemon
- ¼ cup honey
- ¼ teaspoon garlic powder
- 1 teaspoon dried rosemary
- salt

- pepper

Directions:

1. Preheat oven to 400 degrees F.
2. Take a bowl and toss the kale with some salt, pepper, and olive oil.
3. Lightly oil a baking sheet and add the kale.
4. Roast in the oven for 5 minutes, and then remove and place to the side.
5. Place beets in a bowl and sprinkle with a bit of rosemary, garlic powder, pepper, and salt; ensure beets are coated well.
6. Spread the beets on the oiled baking sheet, place on the middle rack of your oven, and roast for 45 minutes, turning twice.
7. Make the lemon vinaigrette by whisking all of the listed in a bowl. Once the beets are ready, remove from the oven and allow it to cool.
8. Take a medium-sized salad bowl and add kale, onions, and beets.
9. Dress with lemon honey vinaigrette and toss well. Garnish with toasted almonds. Enjoy!

Nutrition: Calories: 245, Total Fat: 17.6 g, Saturated Fat: 2.6 g, Cholesterol: 0 mg, Sodium: 77 mg, Total Carbohydrate: 22.9 g, Dietary Fiber: 3 g, Total Sugars: 17.7 g, Protein: 2.4 g, Vitamin D: 0 mcg, Calcium: 50 mg, Iron: 1 mg, Potassium: 416 mg

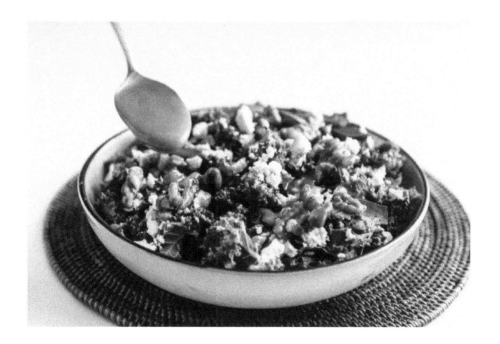

Moroccan Fish

Preparation Time:

5 minutes

Cooking Time:

1 Hour 25 Minutes

Servings: 12

Ingredients:

- Garbanzo beans (15 oz. Can)
- Red bell peppers (2)
- Large carrot (1)
- Vegetable oil (1 tbsp.)
- Onion (1)
- Garlic (1 clove)
- Tomatoes (3 chopped/14.5 oz can)
- Olives (4 chopped)
- Chopped fresh parsley (.25 cup)
- Ground cumin (.25 cup)
- Paprika (3 tbsp.)
- Chicken bouillon granules (2 tbsp.)
- Cayenne pepper (1 tsp.)
- Salt (to your liking)
- Tilapia fillets (5 lb.)

Directions:

1. Drain and rinse the beans. Thinly slice the carrot and onion. Mince the garlic and chop the olives.

2. Discard the seeds from the peppers and slice them into strips.

3. Warm the oil in a frying pan using the medium temperature setting. Toss in the onion and garlic. Simmer them for approximately five minutes.

4. Fold in the bell peppers, beans, tomatoes, carrots, and olives.

5. Continue sautéing them for about five additional minutes.

6. Sprinkle the veggies with the cumin, parsley, salt, chicken bouillon, paprika, and cayenne.

7. Stir thoroughly and place the fish on top of the veggies.

8. Pour in water to cover the veggies.

9. Lower the heat setting and cover the pan to slowly cook until the fish is flaky (about 40 min)

Nutrition: Calories: 268; Protein: 42 grams; Fat: 5 grams

Niçoise-inspired Salad With Sardines

Preparation Time:

5 minutes

Cooking Time:

15 Minutes

Servings: 4

Ingredients:

- 4 eggs
- 12 ounces baby red potatoes (about 12 potatoes)
- 6 ounces green beans, halved
- 4 cups baby spinach leaves or mixed greens
- 1 bunch radishes, quartered (about 1⅓ cups)
- 1 cup cherry tomatoes
- 20 kalamata or niçoise olives (about ⅓ cup)
- 3 (3.75-ounce) cans skinless, boneless sardines packed in olive oil, drained
- 8 tablespoons Dijon Red Wine Vinaigrette

Directions:

1. Place the eggs in a saucepan and cover with water.

2. Bring the water to a boil. As soon as the water starts to boil, place a lid on the pan and turn the heat off. Set a timer for minutes.

3. When the timer goes off, drain the hot water and run cold water over the eggs to cool. Peel the eggs when cool and cut in half.

4. Prick each potato a few times with a fork.

5. Place them on a microwave-safe plate and microwave on high for 4 to 5 minutes, until the potatoes are tender. Let cool and cut in half.

6. Place green beans on a microwave-safe plate and microwave on high for 1½ to 2 minutes, until the beans are crisp-tender. Cool.

7. Place 1 egg, ½ cup of green beans, 6 potato halves, 1 cup of spinach, ⅓ cup of radishes, ¼ cup of tomatoes, olives, and 3 sardines in each of 4 containers.

8. Pour 2 tablespoons of vinaigrette into each of 4 sauce containers.

STORAGE : Store covered containers in the refrigerator for up to 4 days.

Nutrition: Total calories: 450; Total fat: 32g; Saturated fat: 5g; Sodium: 6mg; Carbohydrates: 22g; Fiber: 5g; Protein: 21g

Lettuce Tomato Salad

Preparation Time:

5 minutes

Cooking Time:

15 Minutes

Servings: 6

Ingredients:

- 1 heart of Romaine lettuce, chopped
- 3 Roma tomatoes, diced
- 1 English cucumber, diced
- 1 small red onion, finely chopped
- ½ cup curly parsley, finely chopped
- 2 tablespoons virgin olive oil
- lemon juice, ½ large lemon
- 1 teaspoon garlic powder
- salt
- pepper

Directions:

1. Add all ingredient to a large bowl.
2. Toss well and transfer them to containers.
3. Enjoy!

Nutrition: Calories: 68, Total Fat: 9 g, Saturated Fat: 0.8 g, Cholesterol: 0 mg, Sodium: 7 mg, Total Carbohydrate: 6 g, Dietary Fiber: 1.5 g, Total Sugars: 3.3 g, Protein: 1.3 g, Vitamin D: 0 mcg, Calcium: 18 mg, Iron: 1 mg, Potassium: 309 mg

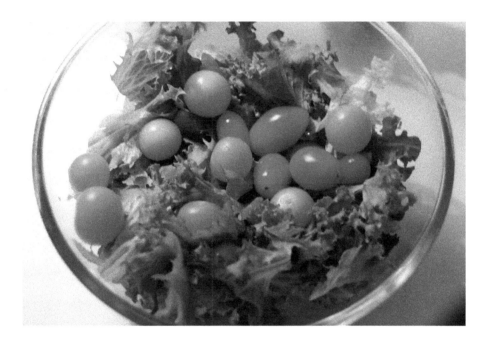

Mediterranean Chicken Pasta Bake

Preparation Time:

5 minutes

Cooking Time:

30 Minutes

Servings: 4

Ingredients:

- Marinade:
- 1½ lbs. boneless, skinless chicken thighs, cut into bite-sized pieces*
- 2 garlic cloves, thinly sliced
- 2-3 tbsp. marinade from artichoke hearts
- 4 sprigs of fresh oregano, leaves stripped
- Olive oil
- Red wine vinegar
- Pasta:
- 1 lb whole wheat fusilli pasta
- 1 red onion, thinly sliced
- 1 pint grape or cherry tomatoes, whole
- ½ cup marinated artichoke hearts, roughly chopped
- ½ cup white beans, rinsed + drained (I use northern white beans)
- ½ cup Kalamata olives, roughly chopped

- ⅓ cup parsley and basil leaves, roughly chopped
- 2-3 handfuls of part-skim shredded mozzarella cheese
- Salt, to taste
- Pepper, to taste
- Garnish:
- Parsley
- Basil leaves

Directions:

1. Create the chicken marinade by drain the artichoke hearts reserving the juice
2. In a large bowl, add the artichoke juice, garlic, chicken, and oregano leaves, drizzle with olive oil, a splash of red wine vinegar, and mix well to coat
3. Marinate for at least 1 hour, maximum hours
4. Cook the pasta in boiling salted water, drain and set aside
5. Preheat your oven to 42degrees F
6. In a casserole dish, add the sliced onions and tomatoes, toss with olive oil, salt and pepper. Then cook, stirring occasionally, until the onions are soft and the tomatoes start to burst, about 15-20 minutes

7. In the meantime, in a large skillet over medium heat, add 1 tsp of olive oil

8. Remove the chicken from the marinade, pat dry, and season with salt and pepper

9. Working in batches, brown the chicken on both sides, leaving slightly undercooked

10. Remove the casserole dish from the oven, add in the cooked pasta, browned chicken, artichoke hearts, beans, olives, and chopped herbs, stir to combine

11. Top with grated cheese

12. Bake for an additional 5-7 minutes, until the cheese is brown and bubbling

13. Remove from the oven and allow the dish to cool completely

14. Distribute among the containers, store for 2-3 days

15. To Serve: Reheat in the microwave for 1-2 minutes or until heated through.

16. Garnish with fresh herbs and serve

Nutrition: Calories: 487; Carbs: 95g; Total Fat: 5g; Protein: 22g

Roasted Vegetable Flatbread

Preparation Time:

5 minutes

Cooking Time:

25 Minutes

Servings: 4

Ingredients:

- 16 oz pizza dough, homemade or frozen
- 6 oz soft goat cheese, divided
- ¾ cup grated Parmesan cheese divided
- 3 tbsp chopped fresh dill, divided
- 1 small red onion, sliced thinly
- 1 small zucchini, sliced thinly
- 2 small tomatoes, thinly sliced
- 1 small red pepper, thinly sliced into rings
- Olive oil
- Salt, to taste
- Pepper, to taste

Directions:

1. Preheat the oven to 400 degrees F

Roll the dough into a large rectangle, and then place it on a piece of parchment paper sprayed with non-stick spray

2. Take a knife and spread half the goat cheese onto one half of the dough, then sprinkle with half the dill and half the Parmesan cheese

3. Carefully fold the other half of the dough on top of the cheese, spread and sprinkle the remaining parmesan and goat cheese

4. Layer the thinly sliced vegetables over the top

5. Brush the olive oil over the top of the veggies and sprinkle with salt, pepper, and the remaining dill

6. Bake for 22-25 minutes, until the edges are medium brown, cut in half, lengthwise

7. Then slice the flatbread in long 2-inch slices and allow to cool.Distribute among the containers, store for 2 days

8. To Serve: Reheat in the oven at 375 degrees for 5 minutes or until hot. Enjoy with a fresh salad.

Nutrition: Calories: 170; Carbs: 21g; Total Fat: 6g; Protein: 8g

Steak Cobb Salad

Preparation Time:

5 minutes

Cooking Time:

15 Minutes

Servings: 4

Ingredients:

- 6 large eggs
- 2 tbsp unsalted butter
- 1 lb steak
- 2 tbsp olive oil
- 6 cups baby spinach
- 1 cup cherry tomatoes, halved
- 1 cup pecan halves
- 1/2 cup crumbled feta cheese
- Kosher salt, to taste
- Freshly ground black pepper, to taste

Directions:

1. In a large skillet over medium high heat, melt butter
2. Using paper towels, pat the steak dry, then drizzle with olive oil and season with salt and pepper, to taste

3. Once heated, add the steak to the skillet and cook, flipping once, until cooked through to desired doneness, - cook for 4 minutes per side for a medium-rare steak

4. Transfer the steak to a plate and allow it to cool before dicing

5. Place the eggs in a large saucepan and cover with cold water by 1 inch

6. Bring to a boil and cook for 1 minute, cover the eggs with a tight-fitting lid and remove from heat, set aside for 8-10 minutes, then drain well and allow to cool before peeling and dicing

7. Assemble the salad in the container by placing the spinach at the bottom of the container, top with arranged rows of steak, eggs, feta, tomatoes, and pecans

8. To Serve: Top with the balsamic vinaigrette, or desired dressing

9. Recipe Note: You can also use New York, rib-eye or filet mignon for this recipe

Nutrition: Calories: 640; Total Fat: 51g; Total Carbs: 9.8g; Fiber: 5g; Protein: 38.8g

Grilled Lamb Chops

Preparation Time:

5 minutes

Cooking Time:

10 Minutes

Servings: 4

Ingredients:

- 4 8-ounce lamb shoulder chops
- 2 tablespoons Dijon mustard
- 2 tablespoons balsamic vinegar
- 1 tablespoon chopped garlic
- ¼ teaspoon ground black pepper
- ½ cup olive oil
- 2 tablespoons fresh basil, shredded

Directions:

1. Pat the lamb chops dry and arrange them in a shallow glass-baking dish.
2. Take a bowl and whisk in Dijon mustard, garlic, balsamic vinegar, and pepper.
3. Mix well to make the marinade.
4. Whisk oil slowly into the marinade until it is smooth.
5. Stir in basil.

6. Pour the marinade over the lamb chops, making sure to coat both sides.

7. Cover, refrigerate and allow the chops to marinate for anywhere from 1-4 hours.

8. Remove the chops from the refrigerator and leave out for 30 minutes or until room temperature.

9. Preheat grill to medium heat and oil grate.Grill the lamb chops until the center reads 145 degrees F and they are nicely browned, about 5-minutes per side.

10. Enjoy!

Nutrition: Calories: 1587, Total Fat: 97.5 g, Saturated Fat: 27.6 g, Cholesterol: 600 mg, Sodium: 729 mg, Total Carbohydrate: 1.3 g, Dietary Fiber: 0.4 g, Total Sugars: 0.1 g, Protein: 176.5 g, Vitamin D: 0 mcg, Calcium: 172 mg, Iron: 15 mg, Potassium: 30 mg

Broiled Chili Calamari

Preparation Time:

5 minutes

Cooking Time:

8 Minutes

Servings: 4

Ingredients:

- 2 tablespoons extra virgin olive oil
- 1 teaspoon chili powder
- ½ teaspoon ground cumin
- Zest of 1 lime
- Juice of 1 lime
- Dash of sea salt
- 1 and ½ pounds squid, cleaned and split open, with tentacles cut into ½ inch rounds
- 2 tablespoons cilantro, chopped
- 2 tablespoons red bell pepper, minced

Directions:

1. Take a medium bowl and stir in olive oil, chili powder, cumin, lime zest, sea salt, lime juice and pepper
2. Add squid and let it marinade and stir to coat, coat and let it refrigerate for 1 hour
3. Pre-heat your oven to broil

4. Arrange squid on a baking sheet, broil for 8 minutes turn once until tender

5. Garnish the broiled calamari with cilantro and red bell pepper

6. Serve and enjoy!

7. Meal Prep/Storage Options: Store in airtight containers in your fridge for 1-2 days.

Nutrition: Calories: 159; Fat: 13g; Carbohydrates: 12g; Protein: 3g

Roasted Beet Salad with Ricotta Cheese

Preparation Time:

10 minutes

Cooking Time:

1 hour

Servings: 4

Ingredients:

- Red beets (8.8 oz, large, wrapped in foil)
- Yellow beets (8.8 oz, small, wrapped in foil)
- Mesclun (4.3 oz)
- Mustard Vinaigrette (4.4 oz)
- Ricotta cheese (2.1 oz)
- Walnuts (0.1 oz, chopped)

Directions:

1. Bake at 400 F until the beets are tender, about 1 hour.
2. Cool the beets slightly. Trim the root and stem ends and pull off the peels.
3. Cut the red beets crosswise into thin slices.
4. Cut the yellow beets vertically into quarters.

5. Arrange the sliced red beets in circles on cold salad plates. Toss the mesclun with half the vinaigrette.

6. Drizzle the remaining vinaigrette over the sliced beets.

7. Place a small mound of greens in the center of each plate.

8. Arrange the quartered yellow beets around the greens.

9. Sprinkle the tops of the salads with the crumbled ricotta and walnuts (if using).

Nutrition: Calories: 290Fat: 6g Carbs: 12g Protein: 6g Fiber: 3g

Baked Fish with Tomatoes and Mushrooms

Preparation Time:

12 minutes

Cooking Time:

25 minutes

Servings: 4

Ingredients:

- Fish (4, whole and small, 12 oz each)
- Salt (to taste)
- Pepper (to taste)
- Dried thyme (pinch)
- Parsley (4 sprigs)
- Olive oil (as needed)
- Onion (4 oz, small dice)
- Shallots (1 oz, minced)
- Mushrooms (8 oz, chopped)
- Tomato concasse (6.4 oz)
- Dry white wine (3.2 fl oz)

Directions:

1. Scale and clean the fish but leaves the heads on. Season the fish inside and out with salt and pepper and put a small pinch of thyme and a sprig of parsley in the cavity of each.

2. Use as many baking pans to hold the fish in a single layer. Oil the pans with a little olive oil.

3. Sauté the onions and shallots in a little olive oil about 1 minute. Add the mushrooms and sauté lightly.

4. Put the sautéed vegetables and the tomatoes in the bottoms of the baking pans.

5. Put the fish in the pans. Oil the tops lightly. Pour in the wine.

6. Bake at 400F until the fish is done. The time will vary but will average 15-20 minutes. Base often with the liquid in the pan.

7. Remove the fish and keep them warm until they are plated.

8. Remove the vegetables from the pans with a slotted spoon and check for seasonings. Serve a spoonful of the vegetables with the fish, placing it under or alongside each fish.

9. Strain, degrease, and reduce the cooking liquid slightly. Just before serving, moisten each portion with 1-2 tbsp of the liquid.

Nutrition: Calories: 350Fat: 9gCarbs: 6g Protein: 55g Fiber: 1g

Goat Cheese and Walnut Salad

Preparation Time:

15 minutes

Cooking Time:

10 minutes

Servings: 3

Ingredients:

- Beet (2 oz)
- Arugula (3 oz)
- Bibb lettuce (2 oz)
- Romaine lettuce (9 oz)
- Breadcrumbs (1/4 cup, dry)
- Dried thyme (1/4 tbs)
- Dried basil (1/4 tbs)
- Black pepper (1/3 tsp)
- Fresh goat's milk cheese (6.35 oz, preferably in log shape)
- Walnut pieces (1.1 oz)
- Red wine vinaigrette (2 fl. Oz.)

Directions:

1. Trim, wash, and dry all the salad greens.
2. Tear the greens into small pieces. Toss well.
3. Mix the herbs, pepper, and crumbs.

4. Slice the cheese into 1 oz pieces. In the seasoned crumbs mix, roll the pieces of cheese to coat them

5. Place the cheese on a sheet pan. Bake at the temperate of 425 F for 10 minutes.

6. At the same time, toast the walnuts in a dry sauté pan or the oven with the cheese.

7. Toss the greens with the vinaigrette and arrange on cold plates.

8. Top each plate of greens with 2 pieces of cheese and sprinkle with walnuts.

Nutrition: Calories: 460 Fat: 40g Carbs: 13g Protein: 17g Fiber: 3

Grilled Spiced Turkey Burger

Preparation Time:

15 minutes

Cooking Time:

20 minutes

Servings: 3

Ingredients:

- Onion (1.8 oz, chopped fine)
- Extra Virgin Olive Oil (1/3 tbsp)
- Turkey (14.4 oz, ground)
- Salt (1/3 tbsp)
- Curry powder (1/3 tbsp)
- Lemon zest (2/5 tsp, grated)
- Pepper (1/8 tsp)
- Cinnamon (1/8 tsp)
- Coriander (1/4 tsp, ground)
- Cumin (1/8 tsp, ground)
- Cardamom (1/8 tsp, ground)
- Water (1.2 fl oz)
- Tomato Raisin Chutney (as desired)
- Cilantro leaves (as desired)

Directions:

1. Cook the onions in the oil until soft. Cool completely.
2. Combine the turkey, onions, spices, water, and salt in a bowl. Toss until mixed.
3. Divide the mixture into 5 oz portions (or as desired). Form each portion into a thick patty.
4. Broil or grill until well done, but do not overcook it, or the burger will dry.
5. Plate the burgers.
6. Place a spoonful of chutney on top of each burger or place it on the side with a small amount of greens.
7. You can serve the burger and garnish as a sandwich on whole-grain bread.

Nutrition: Calories: 250 Fat: 14g Carbs: 2g Protein: 27g Fiber: 1g

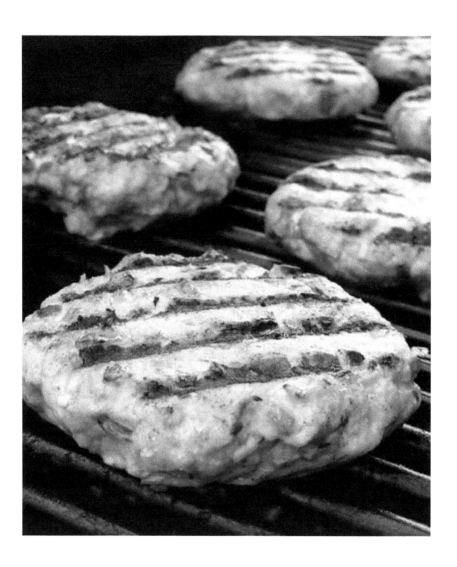

Tomato Tea Party Sandwiches

Preparation Time:

15 minutes

Cooking Time:

10 minutes

Servings: 4

Ingredients:

- Whole wheat bread (4 slices)
- Extra virgin olive oil (4 1/3 tbsp)
- Basil (2 1/8 tbsp., minced)
- Tomato slices (4 thick)
- Ricotta cheese (4 oz)
- Dash of pepper

Directions:

1. Toast bread to your preference.
2. Spread 2 tsp. olive oil on each slice of bread. Add the cheese.
3. Top with tomato, then sprinkle with basil and pepper.
4. Serve with lemon water and enjoy it!

Nutrition: Calories: 239 Fat: 16.4g Carbs: 18.6g Protein: 6g Fiber: 3g

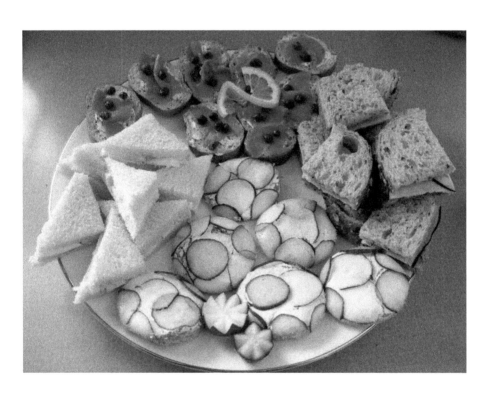

Long-Grain Rice Congee and Vietnamese Chicken

Preparation Time:

10 minutes

Cooking Time:

18 minutes

Servings: 4

Ingredients:

- 1/8 cup uncooked jasmine rice
- 1 whole chicken
- 3 pieces fresh ginger root
- 1 stalk of lemongrass
- 1 tablespoon salt
- 1/4 cup chopped coriander
- 1/8 cup chopped fresh chives
- Ground black pepper to taste
- 1 lime, cut into 8 quarters

Directions:

1. Place the chicken in a pan. Pour enough water to cover the chicken. Merge the ginger, lemongrass, and salt; bring to a boil.

2. Lower the heat, cover, and let it simmer for 1 hour to an hour and a half.

3. Filter the broth and put the broth back in a pan.

4. Allow the chicken to cool, then remove the bones and skin and tear them into small pieces; put aside.

5. Attach the rice to the broth and bring to a boil. Turn the heat to medium and cook for 30 minutes, stirring occasionally.

6. Adjust if congee is done, but you can still cook for 45 minutes for better consistency.

7. Pour the necessary with extra water or salt.

8. The congee into bowls and garnish with chicken, coriander, chives, and pepper.

9. Squeeze the lime juice to taste.

Nutrition: Calories: 642 Fat: 42.3 g Carbohydrates: 9.8 g Protein: 53 g

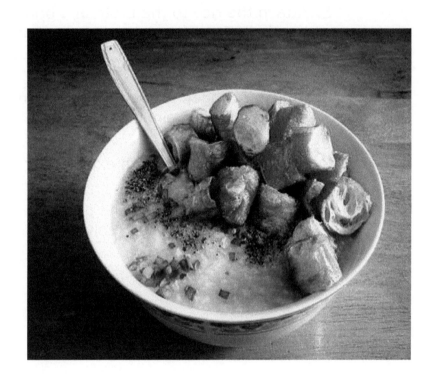

Lightning Source UK Ltd.
Milton Keynes UK
UKHW020825170621
385666UK00005B/80